30 Day Paleo Challenge

The Complete Guide to Lose Rapid Weight by Eating the Foods you Want

By

Nancy Wilson

Table of Contents

Introduction: Getting to Know Paleo

At first glance you might be tempted to discount the Paleo Diet as simply one of many recent weight loss fads, but there is a problem with that assumption; Paleo is not new. In fact, a Paleo Diet of various hues and shades has been employed somewhere on this planet for the whole estimated 200,000 years of human existence. Long ago, in long forgotten prehistoric times, long before any Egyptian or Sumerian had ever learned to write on a temple wall, man was roaming the wilderness, with nothing but his inborn paleo instinct as his guide.

This instinct drove ancient humanity to live in perfect harmony with the environment, hunting, and gathering food as they went along their way. This original paleo diet of our progenitors facilitated a very mobile lifestyle, moving from place to place as our ancestors followed the herds of animals they hunted. This flexible motility

1

stands in stark contrast to the sedentary life that most of us live today. For most, their routine consists of staying in the same general area, and sometimes even the same seat, for several hours at a time.

It actually wasn't until the convergence of two things that humanity began to head towards the doldrums of the non-active, sedentary life that most of us are familiar with today; and those two things were civilization and farming. These two innovations converged to give humanity vast tracts of land turned into farms, to mass produce food, and in turn have this food protected by the laws of civilization. This made it possible for humanity to safely grow and stockpile food, rather than just hunting and gathering as they went along.

This change in diet had a tremendous effect on us. Eating stored grains and veggies on a daily basis had the effect of increasing inflammation in our bodies, whereas the lithe and uninhibited Paleolithic nomads of yesteryear were as healthy as they could ever be! And even though you are not going to go out and kill a wooly mammoth and gather some grub on the frozen tundra anytime soon, a 30-Day Paleo Challenge can quickly put you on the path of a much more healthy and balanced diet. It's called the "30 Day Paleo Challenge".

And with the special guidelines of this challenge you can recreate the diet of our paleolithic past by eschewing all heavily processed foods. You can cut your carbs, and build your protein. The Paleo diet consists of lean meat, and a specific set of fruits and veggies. Maintain this kind of fare for 30 days you can complete the Paleo Challenge. If this sounds like something you would want to do, then follow along with us in this book as we help you get to know all about Paleo.

Chapter 1: Know what to Eat and what Not to Eat as you go Paleo

This book provides you an exclusive listing of Paleo friendly foods. But beyond the recipes in this book, you should take the time to gain a basic understanding for yourself of what works for Paleo and what does not. Any deviation from a regular daily ritual is going to be difficult. But the best way to stem this difficulty is to plan ahead for any challenging contingencies you may face. And since invariably, the biggest challenge of Paleo is simply knowing what to eat, this chapter we will discuss the finer points of what you should and should not eat as you go Paleo.

Monosaturated Fat

Sometimes referred to as "good fat", monosaturated fat is the kind of fat that is already naturally residing in foods such as avocadoes, nuts, and olive oil. I would like to deliver one special word of advice on olive oil, if I may, however. Olive oil provides a fairly condensed offering of monosaturated fat, and if you are not used to having a large amount of it in your system, try to go easy on it at first. Because as good as olive oil is, for the uninitiated, an overdose of it could lead to severe nausea, headaches, and a whole host of other discomfort.

This actually happened to me when I first started out on the Paleo Diet. At first, I loved the way that olive oil tasted as I began my regimen, so much so in fact, that I began giving myself a double portion in my recipes—big mistake. Because as much as I initially loved the stuff, this high intake soon had me waking up in the middle of the night with severe stomach pains, acid reflux, nausea, and even body aches. At first, I thought it was a case of the flu, but then I realized the real culprit was olive oil intoxication!

Yes! There really is such a thing! If you end up ingesting more olive oil than your little digestive organs can handle, then you are intoxicated from it. And for the next 24 hours I felt like I had the worst hangover of my life. That's why in this book we always take care to use a condensed monosaturated fat filled substance such as olive oil, only in moderation. But now that I have thoroughly scared you with my bad run in with monosaturated fat, let me assure you that the benefits that can be gleaned from it, far outweigh the bad.

Doctors everywhere have cited monosaturated fats to play a pivotal role in reducing the onset of cholesterol and they have even been shown to help clear up clogged arteries. These are all incredible benefits of monosaturated fat, and have all been proven, recorded, and documented by the "American Heart Association." Monosaturated fats in moderation have also proven their worth in weight loss, especially in the worst kind of fat accumulation—belly fat. So, all in all a little monosaturated fat is good for you, and many of the recipes in this book have their share of monosaturated fat, just make sure you partake of it in moderate amounts.

Saturated Fat

While monosaturated fat is hailed in the diet and exercise world as the best thing since Richard Simmons, its cousin "saturated fat" on the other hand is a leading cause of cholesterol and weight gain. And this is most certainly bad news for most of us trying t maintain good health A diet high in saturated fat can lead to a whole host of problems. In fact, the only form of saturated fat that is for our benefit is the sat-fat known as "stearic acid".

Unlike its harmful brethren, this highly specialized fat, has the unique ability not only to lower our cholesterol, and facilitate weight loss, stearic acid also serves the unique purpose of helping to improve lung function. You see, the surface of human lung tissue, under optimal conditions, is supposed to be naturally lined with "lung surfactant". It is this lubricating layer of fat, lipids, and protein that allows for better functionality of lung tissue.

If you have asthma, and general tightness of the chest for example, a steady diet of this form of saturated fat, very well could help to open up your breathing passages. Beef, pork, and lamb all have good amounts of stearic acid. And this book provides several variations of these recipes, in order to bring you the kind of nutrition that you need for optimal health.

Polyunsaturated Fat

It is fish at provides us with the most polyunsaturated fat in the form of "omega 3". Omega 3 is quite popular these days and if you go to any health food store or vitamin shop you will see stack upon stack of containers full of omega 3 capsules. Omega 3 has been shown to better facilitate metabolism, and even works to prevent heart disease. Another good polyunsaturated fat beneficial to paleo is "omega 6" which works in much the same way as well. Highlighting the importance of polyunsaturated fat, this book contains a whole chapter devoted to seafood recipes which are completely rich in this much needed resource.

Lean Natural Meat

The best meat you could ever possibly eat while on the paleo diet is grass fed meat. This variety of meat since it is produced all naturally, is free of the hormones and harmful additives commonly found in most store-bought meat. Most fresh water fish—not fish raised in a fish farm—should be free of hormones and additives as well. Lean natural meat plays a pivotal role in the Paleo Diet. Here are some examples of paleo friendly meat that you should try:

- Shrimp
- Halibut
- Beef Heart
- Steamed Clams

- Lean Pork Chops

- Lean Beef Flank Steak

- Lean Pork Tenderloin

- Skinless Turkey Breast

- Skinless Chicken Breast

Stock up on Your Veggies and Fruit

In the paleolithic past people foraged all kinds of fruit and vegetables that were just naturally growing in the environment. No one was farming and planting seeds — at least intentionally—nope, back in those paleolithic heydays plants only grew when mother nature told them to. And Paleo man was simply the wandering beneficiary of this tremendous, natural bounty. It is said that about 50% of all of our Paleolithic ancestor's calories came from these massive foraging runs.

For most of us today however, we simply have other more pressing matters to attend to than roaming around a forest picking berries, cherries, acorns, and digging up roots. The easiest solution to this dilemma is to simply go to a health food store and purchase our fruit and veggie content right off the shelf. Even if we could buy all of our foraged food from the store however, we would still have a hard time consuming the bulky amount of these foods that our ancestors did.

That's why the Paleo diet allows some leeway with this aspect of the regimen. You don't have to kill yourself trying to make half of your caloric intake fruits and veggies. For the purpose of the 30-Day Paleo Challenge a more scaled down version should be sufficient. Here is a listing of some of the best veggies and fruits for you to consume:

- Figs
- Kiwi
- Plums
- Carrots
- Lemon

- Mango
- Cherries
- Papaya
- Grapefruit
- Eggplant
- Cucumber
- Raspberries
- Artichoke
- Tomatillos
- Pomegranate
- Green Onions
- Brussels Sprouts
- Mustard Greens
- Habanero Peppers

Don't Eat Cereal Grain

Don't get me wrong, many cereal grains are low in fat, but they are just not a reliable source of nutrition. In fact, the animals that consume this type of cereal grain will in turn produce unhealthy meat, lacking in proper nutrition as well. This is precisely why we have stressed using nothing but grass-fed meat. There are much more healthy grains that you can consume other than heavily processed cereal grain however. Here is a brief listing of them:

- Buckwheat
- Wild Rice
- Amaranth
- Sorghum
- Quinoa
- Barley
- Millet
- Wheat
- Corn
- Oats
- Rice
- Rye

Eat Nuts but Not Legumes

You may have heard before that peanuts are in fact, *not nuts.* This is 100% correct. Although someone, somewhere along the way, decided to call them "nuts", they are actually "legumes". And that being said, make sure that you cross "peanuts" right off of your list right now. The reason why paleo spurns legumes is due to the fact that they contain lectin and phytic acid which bind to and block important minerals in our bloodstream.

At any rate, you need to avoid legumes such as the—nut in name only—peanut, and only eat real nuts instead. And before you find yourself *going really nuts* after trying to sort all of this all out, trying to sort all of this out in a couple of paragraphs. Allow me to help you by listing the actual nuts that you *can eat,* on the Paleo Diet. Feel free to eat the following nuts:

- Cashews
- Pecans

- Hazelnuts

- Chestnuts

- Brazil nuts

- Macadamia Nuts

- Almonds

- Pistachios

- Pine Nuts

- Walnuts

- Sesame Seeds

- Pumpkin Seeds

- Sunflower Seeds

Dairy to be Avoided

If milk and cheese are some of your favorite foods, I apologize in advance for being the harbinger of bad news. But our paleolithic predecessors didn't eat processed dairy products any more than they ate any other processed food. As tasty as we may think it all is, the second we put this heavily processed food into our body it does quite a number on us, raising our cholesterol, and causing us all kinds of heart and digestive problems, as well as causing us to gain weight. So sadly, enough folks, all of your dairy based cheese, yogurts, and milk shakes will need to be avoided.

Be Mindful of Dining Outside

When you are engaged in a diet as food specific as paleo, you can find yourself hard pressed to find proper Paleo alternatives in short order. It is for this reason that it is recommended to avoid dining out during the first 30 days of the Paleo Challenge. But since social gathering often overrule such inhibitions, you just might find it necessary to have to think on the spot, and surmise the best combination of ingredients that are available for you. The safest route would probably to get a simple salad, minus the dressing and other extras.

But don't be afraid to experiment and ask your server plenty of questions. The more you ask, the more you found out. And in many cases, there are accommodations and recommendation that you wouldn't know anything about, unless you ask. So, don't be afraid to state your case to your servers, bistro's and chef's! They are there to help you after all, and most of them are more than happy to do so. Just a few things that you need to know, before you go Paleo.

Chapter 2: Recipes for your Paleo Breakfast

Breakfast is the most important meal of the day. There isn't much of an argument that can be made against that statement. Multiple studies have shown that how and when we first kickstart the metabolic processes of our body upon reaching wakefulness, can be a determinant factor in how well we function. And this is even more pertinent during your 30-Day Paleo Challenge. You are going to need just the right number of vitamins, protein, and minerals, to get yourself up and going. So, go ahead and feast your eyes on these tasty Paleo recipes for breakfast success!

Apple Cider Paleo Donuts

This recipe is reminiscent of the hot apple cider we so often see in the Fall and Winter months at local cafes and restaurants. Apple Cider is aromatic and satisfying with its rich flavor. This recipe condenses all of that aromatic and flavorful goodness into hot, warm donuts that are just as good for your waist as they are to the taste! These Paleo Donuts will put you in a good mood the very moment you bite into them! And since their made with coconut flour, and other fully approved Paleo ingredients they won't break your Paleo bank in the slightest!

Prep Time: 10 min

Passive Time: 5 min

Cook Time: 4 min

Total Time: 19 min

Here are the exact ingredients:

½ cup of coconut flour

½ teaspoon of cinnamon

½ teaspoon of baking soda

1/8 teaspoon of Celtic sea salt

2 eggs

¼ cup of honey

¼ cup of coconut oil

½ cup of warm cider

¼ cup of ghee

Instructions:

For this recipe you will need a donut maker. So, if you do have one, go ahead and get your donut maker out, and for the moment set it to the side. Now you can get out a small sized mixing bowl and add your ½ teaspoon of cinnamon, your $^{1/8}$ teaspoon of Celtic sea salt. Now get another bowl and add your 2 eggs, ¼ cup of coconut oil, and ½ cup of warm cider.

Take your small bowl of powder ingredients and dump them into your larger mixing bowl of ingredients and stir well. After mixing, scoop up a small batch of batter and deposit it in into your donut cooker. Shut the cooker and cook for about 4 minutes. Serve when ready.

Nutritional Information per Serving

Calories: 201

Total Fat: 6 g

Saturated Fat: 2 g

Cholesterol: 31 mg

Total Carbs: 33 g

Breakfast Bread

Bread is typically a heavily processed grain food, but thanks to this recipe, this Breakfast bread is all Paleo. Made from a blend of vanilla powder, almond butter, and other Paleo friendly ingredients, you can have this tasty, fresh bread for breakfast without any problem! You'll absolutely love the fluffy texture of this Breakfast Bread. And its quick and easy to make. In just a little over a half hour you can whip a batch of some of the best bread this side of the Paleolithic Era!

Prep Time: 5 min

Passive Time: 5 min

Cook Time: 25 min

Total Time: 35 min

Here are the exact ingredients:

1 cup of roasted almond butter

1 tablespoon of honey

¼ cup of vanilla powder

4 eggs

Instructions:

To get started, set your oven to 160 degrees and place your ¼ cup of coconut oil in the loaf tin, and add some baking paper to the bottom of it. Now get out a medium sized mixing bowl and add your cup of almond butter, your 4 eggs, your tablespoon of honey, your ¼ cup of vanilla powder. Get out a hand mixer and use it to thoroughly beat these ingredients together. Next pour ingredients into loaf tin until the batter is uniformly distributed. Put the tin in the oven and allow it to bake for 25 minutes. Take the tin out of the oven and allow it to cool for about 5 minutes. Enjoy your Breakfast Bread!

Nutritional Information per Serving

Calories: 617

Total Fat: 26 g

Saturated Fat: 3 g

Cholesterol: 0 mg

Total Carbs: 68 g

Coconut Flour Paleo Pancakes

Pancakes are an all-time favorite when it comes to breakfast, and thanks to these Coconut Flour Paleo Pancakes, you don't have to be the least bit deprived! Made out of coconut flour, these pancakes have a great taste and go well with just about anything. Eat it as a standalone or as a side, either way you will be in for a good morning ride! The next time you need a good breakfast, just make yourself a batch of these Coconut Flour Paleo Pancakes!

Prep Time: 5 min

Passive Time: 0 min

Cook Time: 5 min

Total Time: 10 min

Here are the exact ingredients:

2 tablespoons of extra virgin olive oil

¼ cup raw honey

¼ cup coconut milk

½ tsp vanilla extract

¼ cup coconut flour

¼ tsp cream of tartar

¼ tsp baking soda

¼ tsp sea salt

3 eggs

Instructions:

First, take your 2 tablespoons of olive oil, your ¼ cup of raw honey, and your 3 eggs, and stir them all together.

Next, add your coconut milk, and your ½ tsp of vanilla extract. Stir these together until they are completely blended. Now add your ¼ cup of coconut flour, your ¼ tsp of cream of tartar, your ¼ tsp of baking powder, and your ¼ tsp of sea salt, and stir these together as well. Dump a small amount of this batter into a crepe pan, and place the pan on medium heat. Cook the pancake for about 5 minutes on each side and serve when ready.

Nutritional Information per Serving

Calories: 31.5

Total Fat: 1.4 g

Saturated Fat: 0.7 g

Cholesterol: 37.2

Total Carbs: 2.2 g

Paleo Breakfast Sandwich

I love sandwiches, and breakfast time is no different. It's great to be able to load up some Paleo friendly bread with all of your favorite breakfast fillings! This breakfast sandwich has bacon, chopped onion, garlic and mayo. Here you just might find the makings of a perfect morning. And even if you can't make anything else, at least make yourself one heck of a sandwich—a Paleo Breakfast sandwich!

Prep Time: 5 min

Passive Time: 30 min

Cook Time: 35 min

Total Time: 1 hour and 20 min

Here are the exact ingredients:

5 pieces of bacon

¼ cup of coconut oil

1 cup of chopped onion

2 cups of chopped spinach

1 tablespoon of garlic powder

¼ cup of maple mayo

1 cup of almond flour

½ cup of tapioca flour

½ tsp of baking soda

¼ cup of coconut flour

2 tablespoons of bacon fat

2 eggs

Instructions:

Set your oven to 350 degrees. Now get out a baking sheet and line it with foil. Evenly lay out your 5 strips of bacon upon this baking sheet and place it in the oven. Allow it to cook for about 15 minutes. While your bacon is cooking get out a medium sized mixing bowl and add your cup of almond flour, 2 of your eggs, and your 2 tablespoons of bacon fat. Stir these ingredients together well, before putting your mixing bowl in the refrigerator.

Allow the mixture to sit in the fridge for about 30 minutes. Once the 30 minutes have passed, take out an additional baking sheet and line it with parchment paper. Now, take out a large spoon and use it to place clumps of batter onto the baking sheet. You should be able to make

5 or 6 biscuits out of these clumps of batter. Place these into the oven and cook for 15 minutes. While your biscuits are cooking, get out a sauté pan and place it on a burner set to medium heat.

Now add your ¼ cup of coconut oil to the pan, allowing it to evenly distribute across the bottom of the pan. Follow this by adding your cup of chopped onions, 1 tablespoon of garlic powder, and your 2 cups of chopped spinach. Allow these to cook for about 5 minutes. Once everything has been cooked, take out your biscuits, cut them open, and deposit your bacon, spinach, egg, and onion mixtures inside. Finally, top it all off by sprinkling your ¼ cup of maple mayo on top, and this Paleo Breakfast Sandwich is complete!

Nutritional Information per Serving

Calories: 284

Total Fat: 18 g

Saturated Fat: 10 g

Cholesterol: 150 mg

Total Carbs: 12 g

Breakfast Crab Cakes

If you ever find yourself feeling a bit crabby when you wake up in the morning, these Breakfast Crab Cakes will snap you right out of it! Made with fresh crab meat cooked in coconut oil, and garnished with mayo and Dijon mustard, the flavor of these lovely little cakes just *pop* right in your mouth. And believe me, once you start eating them, you *can't stop popping them in your mouth!* Give it a try for yourself!

Prep Time: 5 min

Passive Time: 0 min

Cook Time: 10 min

Total Time: 15 mi

Here are the exact ingredients:

1 can of crab meat

¼ cup of coconut oil

2 tablespoons of mayo

1 tablespoon of minced chives

1 tsp of Dijon mustard

½ tsp black pepper

1 tablespoon of sea salt

1 egg

Instructions:

Set your oven to 350 degrees, and grease a baking sheet with ¼ cup of coconut oil. Now get out a medium sized mixing bowl and add the can of crab meat, your 2 tablespoons of mayo, your egg, your 1 tablespoon of minced chives, your 1 tsp of Dijon mustard, your ½ tsp of black pepper and your ¼ cup of sea salt. Mix these ingredients together well. Now take your (clean) hands and use them to shape the ingredients into what will be your "crab cakes". Place each of your crab cakes on your greased baking sheet and insert the pan into the oven. Allow to cook for about 10 minutes. Serve when ready.

Nutritional Information per Serving

Calories: 327

Total Fat: 6 g

Saturated Fat: 0 g

Cholesterol: 0 mg

Total Carbs: 52 g

Paleo Honey and Almond Oats

This recipe is just as tasty as it sounds! Rich and satisfying honey mixed with cinnamon, and sea salt bring on a savory taste that you won't soon forget. And at just 130 calories per serving, this breakfast keeps right on track. With these wholesome Paleo Honey and Almond Oats, you just can't go wrong! Go ahead and make this recipe part of your breakfast plan during your 30-Day Paleo Challenge!

Prep Time: 10 mins

Passive Time: 0 mins

Cook Time: 30 min

Total Time: 40 mins

Here are the exact ingredients:

½ cup of almond pulp

¼ cup of coconut oil

¼ cup of pistachios

1 tablespoon of sesame seeds

2 tablespoons of shredded coconut

3 tablespoons of honey

¼ tsp of sea salt

¾ tsp of cinnamon

½ tsp of vanilla

¼ cup of raisins

Instructions:

Set your oven for 300 degrees. Now get out a large cooking sheet and place your ½ cup of almond pulp onto the pan. Place your sheet into the oven and allow it to cook for about 15 minutes. Now turn the oven temperature up to 325 degrees. Take the cooking sheet out and allow the pulp to cool. Add your ¼ cup of pistachios, your 1 tablespoon of sesame seeds, your 2 tablespoons of shredded coconut, your ¼ tsp of sea salt, and your ¾ cup of cinnamon to the pan and mix them together with the pulp.

Now place back in the oven. Get out a separate bowl and add your 3 tablespoons of honey, ½ tsp of vanilla, and your ¼ cup of coconut oil. Mix these together well and then pour them on top of your ingredients on the cooking sheet. Place the sheet back in the oven and allow it to cook for another 15 minutes. After your 15 minutes are up, allow to cool and your Paleo Honey and Almond Oats are ready to be served.

Nutritional Information per Serving

Calories: 130

Total Fat: 2 g

Saturated Fat: 0 g

Cholesterol: 0 g

Total Carbs: 26 g

Paleo Burrito Breakfast

If you need a pick me up in the morning, this recipe has it! Do you like burrito's? Well then you are in luck my friends, because this Paleo Burrito Breakfast comes fully loaded with spinach, green peppers, black olives, and tomatoes. And to top it all off, this burrito trades in its tortilla shell for a thick slice of ham! Yes—this recipe gets creative, kicking the traditional, carbohydrate dense, flour based burrito to the curb and replacing it with a piece of thick juicy meat! With all of your favorite breakfast ingredients rolled up in a tasty slice of ham— what's not to love?

Prep Time: 5 min

Passive Time: 0 min

Cook Time: 5 min

Total Time: 10 min

Here are the exact ingredients:

2 eggs

4 slices of ham

¼ cup of chopped spinach

¼ cup of chopped black olives

¼ cup of chopped tomato

¼ cup of chopped green bell pepper

Instructions:

Get out a medium sized pan and add your ¼ cup of chopped spinach, your ¼ cup of chopped black olives, your ¼ cup of chopped tomato, and your ¼ cup of chopped green bell pepper to the pan. Set the pan onto a burner set for high heat and begin to sauté the ingredients. Let them cook for about 5 minutes. Now get out a medium sized mixing bowl and add your 2 eggs to the bowl. Stir these ingredients together before pouring them over your veggies in the sauté pan.

Continue to stir the ingredients as they cook, allowing the eggs to scramble over the other ingredients. Now take your 4 slices of ham and use them as your burrito shells, wrapping the cooked ingredients inside the ham slices. Place these stuffed slices of ham back into the pan, allowing them to cook for just a few more minutes, or until crispy and brown. Serve when ready.

Nutritional Information per Serving

Calories: 85

Total Fat: 0 g

Saturated Fat: 0 g

Cholesterol: 0 mg

Total Carbs: 0 g

Banana Cinnamon Breakfast Rolls

This ingenious recipe lets you wrap up delicious bananas and cinnamon into elegant and stylish breakfast rolls! It does take a little bit of your time to put these treats together—about an hour and 20 minutes total—but they are worth it. Since most of us don't have that much time to cook in the morning however you may need to do bit of pre-meal prep in advance. This meal is perhaps best prepared several hours ahead of time, so you don't have to worry preparing them during the morning rush. Just whip up a batch of these rolls the night before, and you can enjoy them the very next morning!

Prep Time: 10 min

Passive Time: 10 min

Cook Time: 60 min

Total Time: 1 hour and 20 min

Here are the exact ingredients:

3 bananas

¼ cup of cinnamon

1 cup of chopped medjool dates

½ cup of water

¼ cup of vanilla

Instructions:

Set your oven for 250 degrees. Next, get out your three bananas and slice them lengthwise into 3 slices. Lay these out on a greased cooking sheet, and place in the oven. Allow these to cook for about 15 minutes. Now get out a medium sized mixing bowl and add your ¼ cup of cinnamon, your 1 cup of chopped medjool dates, your 1.2 cup o9f water, and your ¼ cup of vanilla. Mix these together well. Now, take a spoon and use it to scoop up your date paste ingredients.

Spread these along the length of your banana slices. Now take your banana slices and roll them together like you would any other kind of cinnamon roll. Place your rolls on your cooking sheet and place them back into the oven, allowing them to cook for about 45 minutes. Once cooked, give them a few minutes to cool, and these Banana Cinnamon Breakfast Rolls are ready.

Nutritional Information per Serving

Calories: 405

Total Fat: 33 g

Saturated Fat: 11 g

Cholesterol: 17 mg

Total Carbs: 31 g

Paleo Breakfast Omelet

Just picture it now--you wake up and smell eggs, raisins, and spices, and your nose leads you down to the kitchen where a delicious breakfast is waiting for you. Just the mere aroma of this Paleo Breakfast Omelet is enough to get you up and moving in the morning. With 3 eggs, and a generation portion of raisins, this breakfast is as tasty as it is filing. And at just 234 calories it doesn't set your diet back in the slightest. Be sure and try this great recipe for your next breakfast!

Prep Time: 2 min

Passive Time: 10 min

Cook Time: 5 min

Total Time: 17 min

Here are the exact ingredients:

1 cup of raisins

3 eggs

1 cup of water

1 tsp of all spice

1 tsp of nutmeg

Instructions:

First, take your cup of raisins and add them to a medium sized saucepan. Follow this up by adding your cup of water and setting the burner on high heat. Cook your raisins for about 3 minutes, before turning the burner off and draining all excess water from your pan. Next, get out a small mixing bowl and add your 3 eggs, 1 tsp of all spice, and your 1 tsp of nutmeg.

Stir these ingredients together well, before pouring them over your cooked raisins. Allow your ingredients to cook for about 2 minutes. Turn your burner off and allow your omelet to soak up the residual heat for about 10 minutes. After this, transfer your omelet to a large plate and serve when ready.

Nutritional Information per Serving

Calories: 234

Total Fat: 9 g

Saturated Fat: 2 g

Cholesterol: 212 mg

Total Carbs: 3 g

Paleo Breakfast Fritters

Fritters are those deep-fried, traditional foods so common in places like the American South. These classic treats have been enjoyed for many generations, but despite their enjoyed taste, the nutritional value of most fried fritters is rather lacking. These Paleo Breakfast Fritters are a different story altogether however. Packed with eggs, sweet potatoes, and zucchini, these Paleo Breakfast Fritters are the healthiest fritters you could ever have this side of heaven!

Prep Time: 5 min

Passive Time: 0 min

Cook Time: 6 min

Total Time: 11 min

Here are the exact ingredients:

½ cup of chopped sweet potatoes

½ cup of chopped carrot

½ cup of chopped zucchini

¼ cup of green peas

¼ cup of almond meal

¼ cup of coconut oil

1 tsp of salt

2 eggs

Instructions:

In a medium sized mixing bowl add your ½ cup of chopped sweet potatoes, your ½ cup of chopped carrots, your ½ cup of chopped zucchini, your ¼ cup of green peas, your ¼ cup of almond meal, your 1 tsp of salt, and your 2 eggs. Stir these ingredients together well, and set the bowl to the side for a moment.

Next, get out a medium sized saucepan and add your ¼ cup of coconut oil to the pan. After doing this, go to your mixing bowl and using (clean) hands (it is the flu season after all), shape your Ingredients into small patties and place them down into the bottom of your saucepan. Cook these for about 3 minutes on each side. Your Paleo Breakfast Fritters are ready!

Nutritional Information per Serving

Calories: 81

Total Fat: 6 g

Saturated Fat: 2 g

Cholesterol: 58 mg

Total Carbs: 5 g

Chapter 3: Paleo Recipes for Your Midday Meal

The Midday meal is one of the most important of the day. And during your Paleo 30 Day Challenge, it is even more important. Here are some great recipes to keep you going in the middle of your daily routine, and help keep you on track for the whole duration of your Paleo 30 Day Challenge.

Spicy Bison Burger

If you feel yourself tempted to make a McDonald's run on your lunch break, just reach for a Spicy Bison Burger instead! This burger comes loaded with bison, sea salt, and fresh basil, all packed onto a Paleo friendly bun! This recipe makes 4 burgers, so you can save one for just about every day of your work week. With these tasty burgers packed in your lunch back, you will be able to conquer your cravings and kick those processed drive thru burgers to the curb! Both nutritious and delicious, the fast food joints just can't compare to this brilliant recipe!

Prep Time: 15 min

Passive Time: 0 min

Cook Time: 20 min

Total Time: 35 min

Here are the exact ingredients:

1 egg

2 tablespoons of olive oil

2 tsp salt-free all-purpose seasoning

¼ tsp sea salt

1 ½ pounds of ground bison

8 large tomato slices

1 tsp of Frank's Red-Hot Sauce (per burger)

Instructions:

Take out a large serving bowl and add your 1 egg, your 2 tablespoons of olive oil, your 2 tsp of salt-free all-purpose seasoning, and your ¼ tsp of sea salt. Mix these ingredients together before adding in your 1 ½ pounds of ground bison. Now take your (clean) hands and use them to shape the mixture into four separate patties.

Throw these patties into a large frying pan and set the burner to high heat. Cook the burgers for about 10 minutes on each side. Add a tsp of Frank's Hot Sauce to each burger. Now take your 8 large tomatoes slices and use them as your hamburger buns, placing your burgers in between them. Your Spicy Bison Burgers are ready!

Nutritional Information per Serving

(For 1 Spicy Bison Burger)

Calories: 533

Total Fat: 39 g

Saturated Fat: 9 g

Cholesterol: 131 mg

Total Carbs: 9 g

Coconut Pork Tenderloin

If you find yourself ravenously hungry in the middle of the day, this hearty helping of Coconut Pork Tenderloin will fill you up without compromising your 30-Day Paleo Challenge. This juicy pork tenderloin has a mouthwatering flavor heavily amplified by its garlic, ginger, and sea salt seasonings. And for all this bursting flavor, for food that is incredibly low in calories and carbs! For the hungry person trying to watch their weight, the Coconut Pork Tenderloin seems to be just what the doctor ordered! So, if you need a meal that's filling for your lunch hour, give this recipe a try!

Prep Time: 15 min

Passive Time: 2 hours

Cook Time: 10 min

Total Time: 2 hours and 25 min

Here are the exact ingredients:

1 and ½ pound, sliced, pork tenderloin

¾ cup of unsweetened coconut milk

2 tablespoons of chopped ginger

¼ cup of chopped garlic

½ tsp sea salt

¼ tsp cayenne pepper

¼ cup of shredded coconut

Instructions:

Take a meat mallet and use it to smash your slices of pork tenderloin until they are about half an inch thick. Put these to the side for the moment and get out a medium sized mixing bowl. Add your ¾ cup of unsweetened coconut milk, your 2 tablespoons of chopped ginger, your ¼ cup of chopped garlic, your ½ tsp of sea salt, and your ¼ cup of shredded coconut. Mix these ingredients together well. Now add your 1 and ½ pounds of sliced pork tenderloin to the bowl.

Cover the bowl and place it into your refrigerator so that it can marinate over the next 2 hours. After your meat has marinated for 2 hours, take it out of the fridge and set it to the side for the moment. Get out a large frying pan and place it onto a burner set to high heat. Now transfer your marinated meat to the frying pan and cook it for about 10 minutes. Briefly allow to cool, and serve!

Nutritional Information per Serving

Calories: 175

Total Fat: 10 g

Saturated Fat: 2 g

Cholesterol: 29 mg

Total Carbs: 3 g

<u>*Paleo Chicken Alfredo*</u>

This refreshing blend of Paleo Chicken Alfredo will bring some much-needed life to the monotony of your midday meal routine. With just a cup of chopped chicken breast, some kelp noodles overlain with garlic, and a few other spices, this Paleo Chicken Alfredo is a real show stopper. So if you need something new, make this recipe for your next lunch hour, and your brown bag carrying coworkers down at the office are sure to be jealous!

Prep Time: 5 min

Passive Time: 0 min

Cook Time: 10 min

Total Time: 15 min

Here are the exact ingredients:

1 cup of chopped chicken breast

1 cup of kelp noodles

½ cup of chopped garlic

¼ cup of olive oil

¼ cup of tarragon

1 cup of cashews

1 tsp of onion powder

1 tsp of sea salt

1 tsp of pepper

1 tsp of paprika

Instructions:

Inside a medium sized saucepan place your ¼ cup of olive oil, your ¼ cup of tarragon, your ½ cup of chopped garlic, and your cup of chopped chicken breast. Follow this by adding your cup of kelp noodles. Set the burner to high heat and allow to cook for about 10 minutes. Now turn off the burner and drain the oil from the pan. With the oil drained add your cup of cashews, your 1 tsp of onion powder, your 1 tsp of pepper, and your tsp of paprika. Stir all of your ingredients together, and serve when ready.

Nutritional Information per Serving

Calories: 375

Total Fat: 19 g

Saturated Fat: 10 g

Cholesterol: 95 mg

Total Carbs: 35 g

Midday Meatloaf

Meatloaf has been a comfort food to many of us over the years, and thankfully for us meatloaf lovers, the Paleo Diet doesn't have any problem with that whatsoever! There are several varieties of this classic dish available for the 30-Day Paleo Challenge, and they are all well within range of our nutritional goals when it comes to calories, fat, and carbohydrates. This recipe will win over your heart even as it helps you score a victory for yourself with Paleo. At just 375 calories, this satisfying meal won't break your caloric budget. Just check out this Paleo prepared, Midday Meatloaf!

Prep Time: 5 min

Passive Time: 2 min

Cook Time: 20 min

Total Time: 27 min

Here are the exact ingredients:

½ cup of chopped zucchini

¼ cup of chopped carrots

¼ cup of peas

½ cup of chopped onions

1 pound of mince meat

¼ cup of Italian herbs

1 tsp of salt

1 egg

Instructions:

Go ahead and preheat your oven for 350 degrees. Add your ½ cup of chopped zucchini, your ¼ cup of chopped carrots, your ¼ cup of peas, your ½ cup of chopped onions, and your pound of mincemeat. Thoroughly stir these ingredients together and set them to the side for a moment. After you have done this, get out a muffin tin and line it with muffin cups.

Deposit a scoop of your meat loaf ingredients into each of your muffin cups. Now sprinkle your ¼ cup of Italian herbs and your tsp of salt on top of each one of these mixtures. Place your muffin tin in the oven and allow to cook for about 20 minutes. Once your 20 minutes have passed, serve when ready.

Nutritional Information per Serving

Calories: 229

Total Fat: 12 g

Saturated Fat: 2 g

Cholesterol: 0 mg

Total Carbs: 4 g

Paleo Beef Stroganoff

Made from beef that was grass fed and free from hormones. This beefy piece of stroganoff couldn't be more Paleo perfect! In about 30 minutes time you can put together a tasty blend of beef, onion, mushrooms, and garlic. All of these powerful ingredients make for a great lunch. Give it a try for yourself! You will be completely amazed!

Prep Time: 5 min

Passive Time: 0 min

Cook Time: 10 min

Total Time: 15 min

Here are the exact ingredients:

¼ cup of olive oil

½ pound of grass fed beef

½ cup of chopped onion

½ cup of chopped mushrooms

¼ cup of chopped garlic

1 tsp of salt

1 tsp of pepper

1 cup of coconut milk

¼ cup of arrowroot

1 cup of kelp noodles

2 cups of water

Instructions:

Get out a medium sized saucepan and place it on a burner set for medium heat. Coat the bottom of the pan with your ¼ cup of olive oil. Next, add your 1/2 pound of beef and your ½ cup of chopped onion to the pan. Stir fry these ingredients for about 5 minutes. Next, add your ½ cup of chopped mushrooms, your ¼ cup of chopped garlic, your tsp of salt, and your tsp of pepper. Thoroughly blend these ingredients together before turning your burner off.

Get out a cooking pot and deposit your cup of kelp noodles, 2 cups of water, and your ¼ cup of arrowroot. Put your burner on high heat, and allow these noodles to cook for about 5 minutes. Drain the water from the pan and transfer your cooked noodles to your other pan of ingredients. Your Paleo Beef Stroganoff is now primed and ready for your satisfaction.

Nutritional Information per Serving

Calories: 500

Total Fat: 15 g

Saturated Fat: 5 g

Cholesterol: 20 mg

Total Carbs: 77 g

Turmeric Braised Beets and Leeks

Nothing beats these beets! This recipe is completely Paleo and completely delicious! If you've never tried some beets braised with turmeric, you don't know what you are missing. This whole recipe is truly priceless. Make sure you try it out for yourself at least once, during your Paleo Challenge! It's easy recipes like this that make those 30 days just fly by!

Prep Time: 10 min

Passive Time: 0 min

Cook Time: 1 hour

Total Time: 1 hour and 10 min

Here are the exact ingredients:

2 leeks

4 golden beets

½ cup of chopped garlic

2 tsp of ground turmeric

1 tsp of ground ginger

1 tsp of kosher salt

¼ cup of lemon juice

2 tablespoon of olive oil

4 chicken drum sticks

4 chicken thighs

½ cup of white wine

Instructions:

Set your oven to 425 degrees. Cut your leeks in half, and then cut them into half-moon shapes. Cut the greens from the beets, rinse them off, and then cut the beets in half, before further cutting them into four sections. Now take out a medium sized mixing bowl, add your 2 leeks, your 4 beets, and your beet greens.

Follow this by adding your ½ cup of chopped garlic, your 2 tsp of ground ginger, your 1 tsp of kosher salt, your ¼ cup of lemon juice, and your 2 tablespoons of olive oil. Stir these ingredients together and then transfer them to a 9 x 13-inch baking dish. Now arrange your 4 chicken drum sticks and 4 chicken thighs on top of this mixture and put it in the oven. Cook for about an hour, and enjoy!

Nutritional Information per Serving

Calories: 390

Total Fat: 11 g

Saturated Fat: 1 g

Cholesterol: 0 mg

Total Carbs: 67 g

Meatless Meatballs

Paleo lets you eat all the meat you want, but just in case you have some vegetarian friends over, you could make them a batch of these Meatless Meatballs! Grated zucchini and all the fixings never tasted better! Even without the met, these Meatless Meatballs will earn your admiration and respect!

Prep Time: 5

Passive Time: 0 min

Cook Time: 30 min

Total Time: 35 min

Here are the exact ingredients:

1 egg

¼ cup of olive oil

¼ cup of chopped garlic

1 cup of grated zucchini

½ tsp kosher salt

1 tsp of black pepper

3 tablespoons of chopped basil

1 cup of Italian seasoned breadcrumbs

Instructions:

Get out a large frying pan and add your ¼ cup of olive oil to the pan. Next, add your ¼ cup of chopped garlic, and place the pan onto a burner set for medium heat. Follow this by adding your cup of grated zucchini, and sprinkle your ½ tsp of kosher salt on top, along with your ¼ cup of black pepper. Now add your zucchini to the pan and allow the mixture to cook for about 10 minutes. After your 10 minutes are up, transfer the contents of your pan to a colander.

Remove any lingering moisture before placing the ingredients into a medium sized mixing bowl, along with your cup of Italian bread crumbs, and your egg. With your (clean) hands, work the mixture into approximately 15 balls. Place these balls onto a cooking sheet, put them into the oven, set the temperature for 375 degrees, and allow them to cook for about 20 minutes. After your 20 minutes are up, your Meatless Meatballs are ready.

Nutritional Information per Serving

Calories: 259

Total Fat: 12 g

Saturated Fat: 0 g

Cholesterol: 52 ng

Total Carbs: 30 g

<u>Stir Fried Broccoli</u>

If you like stir fry—then you are absolutely going to love this Paleo recipe for Stir Fried Broccoli! This dish has just the right blend of olive oil, salt, sugar, and beef broth, marinated ever so slightly with soy sauce! This Stir-Fried Broccoli passes the taste test with flying colors! And at less than 100 calories, this stir fry carries its weight in Paleo gold! Make some room for this delicious Stir Fried Broccoli during your 30 Day Paleo Challenge!

Prep Time: 5 min

Passive Time: 0 min

Cook Time: 5 min

Total Time: 10 min

Here are the exact ingredients:

¼ cup of olive oil

2 cups of chopped broccoli

1 tsp of salt

1 tsp of sugar

1 cup of beef broth

1 tablespoon of soy sauce

Instructions:

Get out a large frying pan and place your ¼ cup of olive oil inside. After setting the burner to high heat place your 2 cups of chopped broccoli, followed by your ¼ cup of sugar and your cup of beef broth. Stir these ingredients together well as they cook over the course of the next 5 minutes. Turn your burner off and add your ¼ cup of salt, followed by your tablespoon of soy sauce. Stir all of your ingredients together one more time, and serve when ready.

Nutritional Information per Serving

Calories: 97

Total Fat: 5 g

Saturated Fat: 1 g

Cholesterol: 22 mg

Total Carbs: 24 g

Turkey Lettuce Lunch Wraps

There is nothing quite like fresh ground turkey, mixed with finely diced onions, and garlic. As soon as you bite into these Turkey Lettuce Wraps, the flavor just explodes into your mouth. If you need a midday Paleo pick me up, these Turkey Lettuce wraps will do the trick! It's simple to make, and even easier to eat! Go ahead and have these Turkey Lettuce Wraps for lunch!

Prep Time: 5 min

Passive Time: 0 min

Cook Time: 5 min

Total Time: 10 min

Here are the exact ingredients:

1 tablespoon of olive oil

½ cup of diced onion

½ cup of diced garlic

1 tsp of ginger

1 tsp of cilantro

1 tablespoon of lemon juice

1 pound of ground turkey

4 leaves of romaine lettuce

Instructions:

Place a small sauce pan on high heat and add your ½ cup of diced garlic, and ½ cup of diced onions. Now drizzle your tablespoon of olive oil on top. Stir these ingredients in the pan, as they cook for about 5 minutes. Once these ingredients are cooked, spread out your romaine leaves onto a large plate, and deposit equal portions of the cooked mixture onto the romaine leaves. Fold the romaine leaves neatly together over the cooked ingredients and your Turkey Lettuce Wraps are complete.

Nutritional Information per Serving

(For each individual wrap)

Calories: 203

Total Fat: 8 g

Saturated Fat: 0 g

Cholesterol: 80 mg

Total Carbs: 7.5 g

Chapter 4: Dinnertime Paleo

At the end of the day when you come home tired and hungry you are going to need a Paleo meal that will fill you up right. Paleo has several such satisfying dinner recipes that allow you to stay well within your dietary budget. In this chapter we will take a look at some of the best Dinnertime Paleo feasts!

Thai Beefy Greens

Ok—you might think that eating salad for dinner just isn't satisfying, but you haven't tried Thai Beef Salad! This salad comes with a whole pound of sirloin steak, making it more like a beef buffet than a bowl of greens! Try this recipe and you won't be disappointed!

Prep Time: 10 min

Passive Time: 1 hour

Cook Time: 10 min

Total Time: 1 hour and 20 min

Here are the exact ingredients:

1 pound of sirloin steak

3 tablespoons of fresh lime juice

2 tablespoons fish sauce

2 tablespoons finely grated, fresh ginger

1 tablespoon of olive oil

2 tsp raw honey

5 cups of chopped leaf lettuce

1 cup of chopped green bell pepper

½ cup of chopped cucumber

½ cup of chopped jalapeno

¼ cup of chopped scallions

¼ cup of chopped mint leaves

¼ cup of cashews

2 tablespoons fresh lime juice

2 tablespoons fish sauce

1 tsp olive oil

1 tsp raw honey

Instructions:

Deposit your pound of sirloin steak into a medium sized mixing bowl. Follow this by adding your 2 tablespoons of lime juice, your 2 tablespoons of fish sauce, your 2 tablespoons of ginger, your tsp of olive oil, and your tsp of raw honey. Put a lid on your bowl and allow it to sit in your refrigerator for an hour. After an hour has passed, set your grill to medium heat. Remove the steak from the mixing bowl and place it on the grill. Allow it to cook for about 5 minutes on each side. Take off grill, and add to your bowl of chopped lettuce. Your Thai Beefy Greens are ready to go!

Nutritional Information per Serving

Calories: 420

Total Fat: 16 g

Saturated Fat: 4.7 g

Cholesterol: 125 mg

Total Carbs: 33 g

Masala Kale Casserole

Masala and kale come together for a lovely casserole! This fantastic mixture of cinnamon, ginger, garlic, and serrano peppers, creates the best possible blend for this Masala Kale Casserole!

Prep Time: 2 min

Passive Time: 0 min

Cook Time: 57 min

Total Time: 59 min

Here are the exact ingredients:

2 tablespoons coconut oil

½ cup of chopped onions

½ cup of chopped serrano peppers

¼ cup of chopped garlic

1 tsp of ground ginger

1 tsp of cinnamon

2 cups of tomato puree

1 can of coconut milk

½ cup of chopped cilantro

1 cup of chopped sweet potatoes

1 cup of chopped kale

¼ cup of pepitas

¼ cup of coconut flakes

¼ cup of chopped cilantro

Instructions:

Get out a large frying pan and add your 2 tablespoons of coconut oil, followed by your ½ cup of chopped onions, and your ½ cup of chopped serrano peppers. Set your burner on high heat and cook these ingredients for about 5 minutes. Next, add your teaspoon of chopped garlic, your teaspoon of ground ginger, your cup of chopped kale, your tsp of cinnamon, your ¼ cup of pepita, your ¼ cup of coconut flakes, and your ¼ cup of chopped cilantro.

Cook these ingredients for about 2 minutes, stirring vigorously as the ingredients cook. Next, add your 2 cups of tomato puree, and can of coconut milk. Lower your burner temperature to low heat and allow to simmer for about 10 minutes. After this, turn off the burner and get out a casserole baking dish. Grease the dish with your 2 tablespoons of coconut oil, before pouring your cup of chopped sweet potatoes into the dish.

Now take your frying pan of ingredients and dump it over your chopped potatoes. Put the dish into the oven, set it for 375 degrees, and bake for about 40 minutes. Once cooked, your ingredients should have risen into a uniform casserole. Feel free to cut the casserole into individual pieces, and serve when ready.

Nutritional Information per Serving

Calories: 462

Total Fat: 44 g

Saturated Fat: 6 g

Cholesterol: 0 g

Total Carbs: 43 g

Creamy Chicken, Bacon, and Broccoli Casserole

Just get a load of this dreamy, Creamy Chicken and Broccoli Casserole. This casserole comes complete with finely chopped broccoli and cauliflower, mushrooms, and juicy chicken breast, and even bacon. All marinated in exquisite coconut milk and chicken broth. You really need to try this recipe!

Prep Time: 5 min

Passive Time: 5 min

Cook Time: 40 min

Total Time: 50 min

Here are the exact ingredients:

1 cup of chopped broccoli

1 cup of chopped cauliflower

½ cup of chopped mushrooms

1 cup of chopped chicken breast

1 cup of coconut milk

½ cup of chicken broth

½ cup of chopped almonds

4 slices of (cooked) bacon

1 tablespoon of coconut oil

1 tsp of sea salt

1 egg

Instructions:

Place a large saucepan onto a burner set for high heat and add your tablespoon of coconut oil, followed by your cup of chopped chicken. Sprinkle your tsp of sea salt on top. Stir and cook for about 10 minutes. Once your ten minutes have passed, turn the burner off and transfer the chicken to a glass baking pan. Follow this by adding your cup of chopped broccoli, cup of chopped cauliflower, and your ½ cup of chopped mushrooms on top of the chicken.

Next, add your ½ cup of chicken broth, your cup of coconut milk, and top it all off with your ½ cup of chopped almonds. Briefly mix these ingredients together before, placing foil over the pan and placing it into the oven. Allow to cook for 30 minutes. Once your 30 minutes are up, take the baking pan out of the oven and allow to cool for 5 minutes. Serve when ready.

Nutritional Information per Serving

Calories: 488

Total Fat: 28.9 g

Saturated Fat: 15.4 g

Cholesterol: 122 g

Total Carbs: 12.3 g

Garlic Zucchini Chicken and Noodles

If you need some healthy yet tasty food for dinner, this Paleolithic dish just won't quit! With zucchini, chicken, noodles, and walnuts, marinated and blended to perfection, you will love the results!

Prep Time: 10 min

Passive Time: 0 min

Cook Time: 5 min

Total Time: 15 min

Here are the exact ingredients:

2 zucchinis

¼ cup of olive oil

¼ cup of chopped garlic

½ cup of chopped walnut

½ tsp sea salt

2 cups of chopped chicken

1 cup chopped green apple

1 tsp of pepper

Instructions:

With a julienne cutter, slice your 2 zucchinis into a series of stringy noodles. Set these to the side for a moment and get out a large frying pan. Add your ¼ cup of olive oil to the pan, and set the burner for high heat. Now add your ¼ cup of chopped garlic, and stir it into the oil as it cooks over the next few minutes. After this, add your freshly sliced zucchini noodles.

Stir and cook the noodles into the mixture over the next couple of minutes as well. Move your cooked ingredients over to a bowl or large plate, and then add your ½ cup of chopped walnuts to the pan, followed by your 2 cups of chopped chicken. Cook and stir together over the next few minutes. Serve whenever you are ready.

Nutritional Information per Serving

Calories: 397

Total Fat: 30 g

Saturated Fat: 17 g

Cholesterol: 128 mg

Total Carbs: 5 g

Chicken Meatball Bowl

This Chicken Meatball Bowl comes loaded with ground chicken, grated ginger, chopped parsnips, and just the right amount of sea salt. In this recipe, it all comes together to bring you the best chicken meatballs you've ever had, one bowl at a time!

Prep Time: 10 min

Passive Time: 0 min

Cook Time: 20 min

Total Time: 30 min

Here are the exact ingredients:

1 ½ cup of chopped parsnips

2 tablespoons of olive oil

12 ounces of ground chicken

2 tablespoons of flaxseed meal

2 tablespoons of snipped cilantro

1 tablespoon of grated ginger

½ teaspoon of sea salt

Instructions:

Take out your slicer and use it to cut your parsnips into noodles. Now get out a medium sized frying pan, put it on a burner set for high heat, and add 1 tablespoons of olive oil. Go ahead and place your freshly cut parsnip noodles into your frying pan. Allow them to cook for about 10 minutes, intermittently stirring the ingredients as they cook. Now get out a separate mixing bowl and add your 2 tablespoons of flaxseed meal, your 2 tablespoons of cilantro, your 1 tablespoon of grated ginger, your 12 ounces of ground chicken, and your ½ tsp of sea salt.

Once these have been deposited, use your (clean) hands to shape these ingredients into meatballs. You should be able to make about 15 of them. Go back to your large frying pan and add another one of your tablespoons of olive oil to the pan. Slather the oil across the pan surface evenly, before depositing your meatballs. Cook on high heat for about 10 minutes, occasionally stirring the meatballs as they cook. Your meatballs are complete.

Nutritional Information per Serving

Calories: 135

Total Fat: 5 g

Saturated Fat: 2 g

Cholesterol: 69 mg

Total Carbs: 7 g

Fried Steak and Mushrooms

This Fried Steak and Mushrooms dish will really make your day! These beef steaks seasoned with crack pepper and sea salt perfectly meld with mushrooms, garlic, and garlic.

Prep Time: 5 min

Passive Time: 10 min

Cook Time: 15 min

Total Time: 30 min

Here are the exact ingredients:

2 boneless beef top loin steaks

½ tsp cracked black pepper

¼ tsp sea salt

1 tsp olive oil

½ cup of chopped mushrooms

1 cup of chopped onions

½ cup of chopped garlic

1 cup of dry red wine

1 cup of beef broth

2 ½ tsp arrowroot

Instructions:

Begin by sprinkling your 2 steaks with your ¼ tsp of sea salt and your ½ tsp of cracked black pepper. Now get out a large frying pan and place it on a burner set for medium heat, depositing your teaspoon of olive oil inside. Follow this by adding your seasoned steaks to the mix, cooking them for about 10 minutes. Now take your steaks out of the pan and place them in a separate container.

Go back to your frying pan and place your ½ cup of chopped mushrooms, your cup of chopped onions, your ½ cup of chopped garlic, followed by your cup of red wine. Turn your burner up to high heat, and cook over the next 5 minutes as you stir vigorously. After 5 minutes have passed, turn your burner off and add your 2 ½ tsp of arrowroot to the pan.

Stir well one final time before putting your steaks down into the pan of ingredients. Cover your pan and let the steaks marinate with the rest of the ingredients for about 10 more minutes. After they are well marinated, serve up these steaks whenever you are ready to do so.

Nutritional Information per Serving

Calories: 267

Total Fat: 11 g

Saturated Fat: 4 g

Cholesterol: 69 mg

Total Carbs: 8 g

Grilled Ribeye Steaks with Smoky Tomatoes

There's nothing better than a little bit of Grilled Ribeye with Smoky Tomatoes. This mix of paprika, sea salt, ground sage, garlic powder, dry mustard, and black pepper, create a perfect flair for this awesome Paleo perfect recipe!

Prep Time: 10 min

Passive Time: 0 min

Cook Time: 25 min

Total Time: 35 min

Here are the exact ingredients:

2 tsp paprika

1 tsp sea salt

½ tsp ground sage

¼ tsp garlic powder

¼ tsp dry mustard

¼ tsp black pepper

4 boneless beef ribeye steaks

7 Roma tomatoes

1 cup of chopped green onions

Instructions:

Get out a small mixing bowl and add your 2 tsp of paprika, your 1 tsp of sea salt, your ½ tsp of ground sage, your ¼ tsp of garlic powder, your ¼ tsp of dry mustard, and your ¼ tsp of black pepper. Mix this together well, before removing 1 tsp of the mix from the bowl and sprinkle it over your 4 boneless beef ribeye steaks. Once your steaks are coated with the mixture, place them on your grill and set the temperature to medium heat.

Allow the steaks to cook for about 10 minutes on each side, before placing them onto a large plate and setting them to the side. Now take another tsp of your spice mixture and sprinkle it over your 7 Roma tomatoes. Place your tomatoes, along with your cup of chopped green onions onto the grill and allow them to cook under medium heat for 5 minutes. Turn off your grill and transfer the tomatoes and onions to the plate with your steak and this paleo dinner is ready to eat!

Nutritional Information per Serving

Calories: 782

Total Fat: 61 g

Saturated Fat: 25 g

Cholesterol: 185 mg

Total Carbs: 8 g

Club Med Steaks

No matter what kind of day you may have had, when you come home for dinner, this recipe will set you completely at ease. You'll feel like you're at Club Med when you eat these steaks!

Prep Time: 10 min

Passive Time: 0 min

Cook Time: 15 min

Total Time: 25 min

Here are the exact ingredients:

¼ cup of lemon juice

7 boneless beef shoulder top blade steaks

1 tsp dried rosemary

¼ tsp sea salt

¼ tsp black pepper

3 tablespoons olive oil

1 cup of chopped brussels sprouts

¼ cup of balsamic salad dressing

2 cups of chopped tomatoes

¼ cup of chopped garlic

¼ cup of pitted green olives

Instructions:

First, take your ¼ cup of lemon juice and sprinkle your steaks with it, followed by your teaspoon of dried rosemary, your ¼ teaspoon of black pepper and your ¼ teaspoon of sea salt. Get out a large frying pan and deposit 1 tablespoon of your olive oil into the pan. Set the burner to high heat, before adding your seasoned steaks to the pan. Let these cook in your pan for about 10 minutes before transferring the steaks to a separate plastic container.

After you have done this, you can add your cup of chopped Brussels sprouts to the pan, followed by your ¼ cup of balsamic salad dressing. Cook these ingredients together over the next 5 minutes. Now go back to your other pan and add your cup of chopped tomatoes, your ¼ cup of chopped garlic, and your ¼ cup of pitted green olives. Stir these ingredients together well. Pour these ingredients over your steaks and they are ready to serve.

Nutritional Information per Serving

Calories: 393

Total Fat: 31 g

Saturated Fat: 6 g

Cholesterol: 56 mg

Total Carbs: 14 g

Paleo Chicken Arugula

Juicy chicken breasts, slathered with olive oil, and garnished with arugula, spinach, and grapefruit. Other chicken recipes pale in comparison to this fine batch of Paleo Chicken Arugula!

Prep Time: 10 min

Passive Time: 0 min

Cook Time: 5 min

Total Time: 15 min

Here are the exact ingredients:

4 chicken breast halves

¼ cup of olive oil

3 cups of arugula

2 cups of shredded fresh baby spinach

1 cup of chopped grapefruit

1 cup of chopped avocado

½ cup of chopped fennel

Instructions:

Make use of the flat side of a meat mallet, to make your 4 chicken breast halves as flat as possible. After you have done this, get out a large frying pan and add your ¼ cup of olive oil, coating the bottom of it, before setting the burner on high. Follow this by adding your 4 chicken breast halves to the pan.

Cook the chicken for about 5 minutes. Now get out a large plate. and place your 3 cups of arugula, 2 cups of shredded baby spinach, your cup of chopped grapefruit, your cup of chopped avocado, and your ½ cup of chopped fennel on top of the plate. Arrange your chicken on top of these ingredients, and serve.

Nutritional Information per Serving

Calories: 314

Total Fat: 11 g

Saturated Fat: 2 g

Cholesterol: 82 mg

Total Carbs: 20 g

Paleo Pork Rhubarb

If you love pork and you love rhubarb, then this recipe is for you! Paleo Pork Rhubarb brings it on home with a whole pound of chopped boneless pork, greatly complimented by rhubarb, chopped onions, and apples, cauliflower couscous, and a healthy amount of chicken broth. Everything you need is right here in this tasty Paleo Pork Rhubarb!

Prep Time: 10 min

Passive Time: 0 min

Cook Time: 10 min

Total Time: 20 min

Here are the exact ingredients:

1 tablespoon of olive oil

1 pound of lean, chopped boneless pork

1 cup of chopped onions

1 ½ cups sliced rhubarb

1 cup of chopped apple

1 cup of chicken broth

2 tablespoons of apple juice

1 tablespoon of sage

2 teaspoons of arrowroot

½ teaspoon of black pepper

1 cup of cauliflower couscous

Instructions:

Get out a large frying pan and place it on a burner set to medium heat. Add your pound of chopped boneless pork to the pan and allow it to cook over the course of the next 5 minutes. After your 5 minutes have passed, transfer your pork from the pan to a separate plastic container. Now add your cup of chopped onions, cup of chopped apple, and your 1 ½ cups of sliced rhubarb to the pan and cook for about 5 minutes, stirring as the ingredients cook.

Take out a small separate bowl and add your cup of chicken broth, your 2 tablespoons of apple juice, your tablespoon of sage, your 2 teaspoons of arrowroot, and your ½ teaspoon of black pepper. Mix these ingredients together well before adding them to your pan. Stir all of these ingredients together as they cook over the course of the next 2 to 3 minutes. Now get out a large plate and deposit your cup of cauliflower couscous onto it. Add your cooked ingredients pork rhubarb ingredients on top and your Paleo Pork Rhubarb is complete.

Nutritional Information per Serving

Calories: 270

Total Fat: 11 g

Saturated Fat: 2 g

Cholesterol: 65 mg

Total Carbs: 16 g

<u>*Sweet Potato Garlic Pork Hash*</u>

Check out this Sweet Potato Garlic Pork Hash! It comes with pork, potato hash, and all the fixings! Give it a try!

Prep Time: 8 min

Passive Time: 0 min

Cook Time: 12 min

Total Time: 20 min

Here are the exact ingredients:

4 cups of chopped sweet potatoes

1 ½ pounds of pork tenderloin

2 tablespoons of sodium beef broth

½ tsp of sea salt

¼ cup of black pepper

3 tablespoons of olive oil

½ cup of chopped garlic

Instructions:

To get started place your 4 cups of chopped sweet potatoes in a medium sized mixing bowl and cover it with some plastic wrap. Put in the microwave and cook for about 8 minutes. Remove from microwave and take off plastic wrap, and set potatoes to the side for now. Get out a large frying pan and deposit your 3 tablespoons of olive oil. Set your burner on high, and add your ½ cup of chopped garlic. Stir your garlic into the oil and cook for about 3 minutes.

After your 3 minutes have passed, transfer cooked onions to a separate container and add your 1 and ½ pounds of pork tenderloin to the pan. Cook your pork for about 5 minutes, before moving the meat out of the pan and into your separate container with your onions. Add your 4 cups of chopped sweet potatoes to the pan and cook for 2 minutes as you stir the potatoes into the oil. Turn off your burner. Spoon this hash out onto a plate, and top with your meat and onion mixture. Your Sweet Potato Garlic Pork Hash is now ready to serve!

Nutritional Information per Serving

Calories: 451

Total Fat: 16 g

Saturated Fat: 3 g

Cholesterol: 107 mg

Total Carbs: 39 g

Chapter 5: Paleo Seafood

Our Paleolithic ancestors loved seafood and I would wager that a great many of you reading this book do as well. So here is a chapter completely dedicated to every paleo friendly fish and crustacean to ever step out of the waters!

Drunk Shrimp on a Stick

Look out everybody because this Paleo seafood is under the influence—the influence of good eating! Drunk Shrimp on a Stick comes completely drenched in lime juice, olive oil, and of course—a batch of 100 percent agave tequila!

Prep Time: 25 min

Passive Time: 15 min

Cook Time: 10 min

Total Time: 45 min

Here are the exact ingredients:

1 pound of sea scallops

12 ounces of large shrimp

¼ cup of 100 percent agave tequila

¼ cup of lime juice

¼ cup of olive oil

2 tablespoons of snipped, fresh oregano

¼ cup of chopped garlic

2 tsp of sea salt

2 tsp of agave syrup

½ tsp of paprika

4 cups chopped jicama

1 cup of chopped avocado

½ cup of chopped cilantro leaves

¼ cup of salt

¼ cup of black pepper

Instructions:

Place your shrimp and scallops in a large plastic bag, and lay it out on a large platter. Get out a small mixing bowl and add your ¼ cup of 100 percent agave tequila, your ¼ cup of lime juice, your ¼ cup of olive oil, your 2 tablespoons of snipped, fresh oregano, your cup of chopped garlic, your 2 tsp of sea salt, your 2 tsp of agave syrup, and your ½ tsp of paprika. After mixing these ingredients together, remove about half of it from the bowl and set to the side for the moment.

Now take what's left of the ingredients in your small mixing bowl and pour them over your shrimp and scallops. Seal the bag back up, and flip it to the other side as you lay it on the platter, to allow the marinade to seep through to the other side of the meat. Repeat this process two or three more times over the course of the next 15 minutes. After you have done this, get out a medium sized mixing bowl and add your 4 cups of chopped jicama, your cup of chopped avocado, and your ½ cup of chopped cilantro leaves to the bowl.

Now take your left-over half of marinade ingredients and pour it on top. Stir this together well, and place in the fridge. Now go to your bag of shrimp and scallops. Open up the plastic bag and drain out the marinade. You can save this for later use, or discard. With your marinade drained from your meat, get out some skewers and place your shrimp and scallops on the skewers, with about ½ an inch between each piece of your meat.

You can now place this seafood over the grill and cook on medium heat for about 10 minutes. Once cooked, serve up this Drunk Shrimp on a Stick with your refrigerated bowl of marinade dipping sauce!

Nutritional Information per Serving

Calories: 306

Total Fat: 11 g

Saturated Fat: 1 g

Cholesterol: 843 mg

Total Carbs: 16 g

Avocado Snapper

Just look at this recipe with its pound of red snapper fillets, cup of chopped avocado, 2 tablespoons of chopped red onion. Just one look, and it becomes perfectly clear, that this Avocado Snapper will get you filled up right!

Prep Time: 10 min

Passive Time: 0 min

Cook Time: 5 min

Total Time: 15 min

Here are the exact ingredients:

1 pound of skinless red snapper fillets

1 cup of chopped avocado

2 tablespoons of chopped red onion

1 tablespoon of snipped cilantro

¼ cup of lime juice

¼ tsp of sea salt

2 tablespoons of olive oil

¼ cup of black pepper

Instructions:

Get out a medium sized mixing bowl and add your cup of chopped avocado, your 2 tablespoons of chopped red onion, your tablespoon of snipped cilantro, your ¼ cup of lime juice, and your ¼ cup of sea salt. Stir these ingredients together and set to the side for the moment.

Now take your fish, rinse them well and cut them into four sections. Coat your fish with your ¼ cup of black pepper. Place your fish in a medium sized frying pan and set the burner on high heat. Cook these fish for about 5 minutes. Pour your separate container of ingredients over the fish as marinade, and get ready to eat!

Nutritional Information per Serving

Calories: 206

Total Fat: 11 g

Saturated Fat: 2 g

Cholesterol: 65 mg

Total Carbs: 4 g

Paleo Poached Fish

Take a whole pound of fresh salmon, some chopped garlic, and honey, and this is precisely how they liked to poach their fish back in Paleolithic times! This is a great recipe to have on hand during your 30 Day Paleo Challenge!

Prep Time: 15 min

Passive Time: 0 min

Cook Time: 1 hour

Total Time: 1 hour and 15 min

Here are the exact ingredients:

1 pound of salmon fillets

¼ cup of chopped garlic

¼ cup of Dijon style mustard

¼ cup of honey

¼ cup of white wine vinegar

¼ cup of dried dill weed

¼ cup of chopped onion

¼ cup of reduced sodium chicken broth

2 pounds of Swiss chard

Instructions:

Start off by rinsing your salmon, and then arranged them down at the bottom of a slow cooker. Now take your ¼ cup of chopped garlic and sprinkle it on top of your salmon fillets. Next, get out a small bowl and add your ¼ cup of Dijon style mustard, your ¼ cup of honey, your ¼ cup of white wine vinegar, and your ¼ cup of dill weed. Mix these together before removing 2 tablespoons of the mixture and sprinkling it over your salmon in the slow cooker.

Put a lid on the remaining mix and set it to the side for the moment. Now go back to your slow cooker, put the lid on it, and set it for a cook time of 1 hour on high heat.

After it has cooked for an hour, take the fish out of the slow cooker and place them onto a large plate or platter. Now take your remaining marinade and drizzle it over the salmon. Your Paleo Poached Fish are ready for some action!

Nutritional Information per Serving

Calories: 287

Total Fat: 9 g

Saturated Fat: 1 g

Cholesterol: 78 mg

Total Carbs: 19 g

Fish and Cabbage Tacos

If you love fish, then you will these Fish and Cabbage Tacos! Check out this lettuce loaded up with halibut, tomatillos, and garlic! You are going to love it!

Prep Time: 30 min

Passive Time: 0 min

Cook Time: 10 min

Total Time: 40 min

Here are the exact ingredients:

1 pound of halibut fillets

½ cup of diced tomatillos

2 tsp of olive oil

¼ cup of chopped garlic

½ tsp of orange zest

½ tsp of lime zest

¼ tsp of sea salt

¼ cup of black pepper

½ cup of chopped lettuce

Instructions:

To get started, thaw out your fish (unless already thawed), and cut them into little pieces, about an inch across. Place your chopped fish into a medium sized mixing bowl followed by your ½ cup of diced tomatillos. On top of these add your teaspoons of olive oil, your ¼ cup of chopped garlic, your ½ tsp of orange zest, your ½ tsp of lime zest, your ¼ tsp of sea salt, and your ¼ cup of black pepper.

Next, heat up your broiler and spread your fish mixture of ingredients onto a large cooking sheet, lightly greased with your remaining tsp of olive oil. Broil these ingredients for about 10 minutes. Once your fish mixture is cooked, place your ½ cup of chopped lettuce at the bottom of a large bowl and then arrange your cooked fish ingredients on top. Your seafood feast is now on the menu!

Nutritional Information per Serving

Calories: 196

Total Fat: 9 g

Saturated Fat: 1 g

Cholesterol: 49 mg

Total Carbs: 7 g

Lemony Tuna Salad

If you need a feel-good meal, this tasty Lemony Tuna Salad is simple to make, and it will put a smile on your face!

Prep Time: 15 min

Passive Time: 0 min

Cook Time: 0 min

Total Time: 15 min

Here are the exact ingredients:

¼ cup of lemon juice

½ cup of chopped fennel

½ cup of chopped red onions

1 package of arugula

2 cans of tuna

1 cup of chopped tomatoes

Instructions:

Take out a medium sized mixing bowl and add your ½ cup of chopped red onions, your ½ cup of chopped fennel, and your ¼ cup of lemon juice. Mix these together well before adding package of arugula, your 2 cans of tuna, and your cup of chopped tomatoes. Stir all the ingredients together one more time, and your Lemony Tuna Salad is ready whenever you are!

Nutritional Information per Serving

Calories: 104

Total Fat: 2 g

Saturated Fat: 1 g

Cholesterol: 24 mg

Total Carbs: 7 g

Spicy Shrimp Fried Cauliflower Rice

Spicy Shrimp Fried Cauliflower Rice! Need I say more? If you love seafood, this Paleo based meal is just what you are looking for!

Prep Time: 15 min

Passive Time: 10 min

Cook Time: 5 min

Total Time: 30 min

Here are the exact ingredients:

2 eggs

8 ounces of frozen shrimp

4 cups of cauliflower florets

1 tsp of toasted sesame oil

1 tablespoon of olive oil

¼ cup of chopped garlic

2 cups of chopped cabbage

1 cup of shredded carrots

½ tsp of sea salt

¼ cup of crushed red pepper

¼ cup of chopped green onions

2 tablespoons of snipped fresh cilantro

Instructions:

Start off by thawing out your frozen shrimp, this should take about 10 minutes at room temperature. While the shrimp are thawing, go to your blender and add your 4 cups of cauliflower florets, and hit the "pulse" button on your blender 2 or 3 times until your cauliflower has been reduced to tiny pieces. Now get out a large frying pan and place it on a burner set for medium heat, before adding your tablespoon of olive oil to the frying pan.

After you have done this, add your 2 eggs to the pan and mix them into the oil as they cook over the next few minutes. Next, place your shrimp in the pan, followed by your ¼ cup of garlic, your 2 cups of chopped cabbage, and your cup of shredded carrots. Stir these ingredients together well as they continue to cook over the next 5 minutes. Allow to cool and serve when ready.

Nutritional Information per Serving

Calories: 180

Total Fat: 7 g

Saturated Fat: 1 g

Cholesterol: 170 mg

Total Carbs: 14 g

Baked Catfish

This tasty morsel will remind you why you like seafood!

The best catfish and spice packed into a casserole dish!

Prep Time: 5 min

Passive Time: 0 min

Cook Time: 20 min

Total Time: 25 min

Here are the exact ingredients:

2 tsp of olive oil

1 tablespoon of garlic powder

¼ cup of lemon juice

1 tsp of black pepper

¼ of a tsp of cayenne pepper

¼ of a tsp of turmeric

1 pound of catfish

Instructions:

Grease the bottom of a casserole dish with 1 tsp of olive oil and place your pound of catfish into the dish. Set this to the side for a moment, and place a small saucepan onto a burner set for medium heat. Into this saucepan add your tablespoon of garlic powder, your tsp of turmeric, your tsp of black pepper, and your remaining tsp of olive oil. Stir these ingredients together as they cook over the next 5 minutes.

After this, turn the burner off, place a lid on the saucepan and go back to your casserole dish of catfish. Drizzle your ¼ cup of lemon juice over the fish, and place the dish in the oven. Set the temp for 420 degrees and allow it to cook for 15 minutes. Once your 15 minutes have passed, turn off your oven, take the casserole dish out and pour the small saucepan of ingredients over your catfish. This Baked Catfish is ready to eat!

Nutritional Information per Serving

(per square)

Calories: 150

Total Fat: 9 g

Saturated Fat: 2 g

Cholesterol: 55 mg

Total Carbs: 5 g

Grilled Salmon

Healthy grilled salmon with just the right blend of spice! This Grilled Salmon recipe is second to none!

Prep Time: 10 min

Passive Time: 0 min

Cook Time: 10 min

Total Time: 20 min

Here are the exact ingredients:

4 salmon fillets

¼ tsp kosher salt

¼ tsp of black pepper

¼ cup of chopped red onion

¼ cup of olive oil

1 tablespoon of balsamic vinegar

1 cup of chopped tomatoes

¼ cup of chopped garlic

¼ cup of chopped basil leaves

¼ cup of dried avocado

Instructions:

Get out a medium sized mixing bowl and add your ¼ cup of dried avocado, your ¼ cup of chopped red onion, your ¼ cup of olive oil, your tablespoon of balsamic vinegar, your ¼ tsp of kosher salt, and your ¼ tsp of black pepper. Mix all of these ingredients together well, and then set the bowl to the side for the moment. Now go to your grill and set it to medium heat. Place your 4 salmon fillets on the grill, close it, and have them cook for about 10 minutes. After this, you can lift the cover and add your avocado mixture on top of your fish. Serve when ready.

Nutritional Information per Serving

Calories: 340

Total Fat: 19 g

Saturated Fat: 2.5 g

Cholesterol: 94 mg

Total Carbs: 7 g

Marinated Shrimp Scampi

This shrimp dish is one of the best Paleo seafood recipes you will ever find!

Prep Time: 35 min

Passive Time: 1 hour

Cook Time: 20 min

Total Time: 1 hour and 55 min

Here are the exact ingredients:

2 pounds of extra jumbo, frozen shrimp

¼ cup of olive oil

¼ cup of dry white wine

¼ cup of chopped garlic

½ tsp crushed red pepper

1 tsp of lemon juice

½ tsp of sea salt

1 tsp of parsley

Instructions:

Unthaw your frozen shrimp, and place them into a large plastic bag. Now get out a medium sized mixing bowl and add your ¼ cup of olive oil, your ¼ cup of dry white wine, your ¼ cup of chopped garlic, your ½ tsp o crushed red pepper, your tsp of lemon juice, and your ½ tsp of sea salt.

Stir these together and pour over your shrimp in the bag. Now seal the bag up and place it in your fridge. Let it marinate in the fridge for about 1 hour. After your hour has passed, drain the liquid out of your bag and place your shrimp in a large frying pan. Set the burner on high and cook for about 20 minutes. Serve when ready.

Nutritional Information per Serving

Calories: 126

Total Fat: 4 g

Saturated Fat: 1 g

Cholesterol: 138 mg

Total Carbs: 2 g

Chapter 5: Paleo Desserts

Even during the paleo challenge you should treat yourself to a dessert every once in a while. Here is a complete listing of several paleo desserts that you can use to lighten your paleo load!

Iced Orange Citrus

If you are fond of the Orange Julius drink you enjoyed back in your Mall Rat days, then you will love drinking this Iced Orange Citrus! It is blended and mixed to perfection, try out this recipe for yourself!

Prep Time: 20 min

Passive Time: 5 hours and 10 minutes

Cook Time: 5 min

Total Time: 5 hours and 35 minutes

Here are the exact ingredients:

1 ½ cup of orange juice

2 tablespoons of agave syrup

1 cup of fresh orange juice

½ cup of fresh lemon juice

Instructions:

Get out a medium sized saucepan and add your 1 and ½ cup of orange juice, followed by your 2 tablespoons of agave syrup to the pan and set the burner for medium heat. Cook for about 5 minutes, before turning off the burner and adding your ½ cup of lemon juice to the pan. Stir all of these ingredients together well before pouring them into a square plastic container. Put this container into your freezer and allow to freeze for about 5 hours. After your 5 hours have passed, allow the mixture to sit at room temperature for about 10 minutes before serving.

Nutritional Information per Serving

Calories: 48

Total Fat: 0 g

Saturated Fat: 0 g

Cholesterol: 0

Total Carbs: 13 g

Ginger Orange Paleo Pears

Ginger Orange Paleo Pears are good for any occasion that comes your way. These tasty pears soaked in orange juice and ginger are a smooth and tasty treat!

Prep Time: 35 min

Passive Time: 2 hours

Cook Time: 0 min

Total Time: 2 hours and 35 min

Here are the exact ingredients:

4 pears

2 cups of fresh orange juice

1 cup of water

1 tsp of cinnamon

1 tsp of chopped ginger

¼ cup of chopped cloves

1 tsp of vanilla

1/8 tsp of nutmeg

Instructions:

Get out your pears and cut about half an inch off the bottoms of each of them. Next, remove the core of the pear but leave the stem in place. Once you have done this, get out a medium sized saucepan, place it on a burner set for high heat, and add your 1/8 tsp of nutmeg, your ¼ cup of chopped cloves, your tsp of cinnamon, your tsp of chopped ginger, your cup of water, and your 2 cups of orange juice.

Stir all of these ingredients together well and let them cook for about 5 minutes. After 5 minutes have passed, add the pears to the pan, lower your burner to "low heat" and allow them to cook with the rest of the ingredients for about 15 minutes. Finally, turn the burner off, and remove your pan from the burner. Add your teaspoon of vanilla, and stir everything together as the ingredients cool.

Empty the contents of your pan into a large plastic container. Cover the container and place in your refrigerator. Once the pear mixture has chilled for about 2 hours and 30 minutes, take out of the fridge, scoop up into bowls, and serve.

Nutritional Information per Serving

Calories: 78

Total Fat: 0 g

Saturated Fat: 0 mg

Cholesterol: 0 mg

Total Carbs: 20 g

Coconut Coffee Ice Cream with Almonds

Do you like coffee? Well—what about ice cream? Then you are in luck! Because this incredible Paleo recipe has married the two like never before! With a full cup of coconut milk mixed with ice water, vanilla, honey, and espresso, you can stay alert and wide awake, with a good taste in your mouth!

Prep Time: 35 min

Passive Time: 4 hours

Cook Time: 0

Total Time: 4 hours and 35 min

Here are the exact ingredients:

1 cup of unsweetened coconut milk

1 cup of ice water

1 vanilla bean

2 tsp instant espresso coffee powder

¼ cup of honey

6 eggs

Instructions:

First, get out your cup of coconut milk and pour it into a large saucepan. Next, cut your vanilla bean lengthwise and empty out all of the seeds into your coconut milk. Set your burner for medium-high heat and cook these ingredients for 5 minutes. Now add your 2 teaspoons of espresso coffee powder, and your ¼ cup of honey into your milk. Lower your burner to "low heat" and stir the ingredients as they simmer together over the next few minutes.

Turn your burner off, and get out a medium sized mixing bowl. Add your 6 eggs and vigorously stir them together. Once the eggs are mixed together slowly pour in 2 cups of your coconut milk from the saucepan, into the mixing bowl. After stirring these ingredients together, transfer them back to the saucepan. Set the burner to medium and stir the ingredients as they cook over the next 5 minutes.

Now get out a separate plastic container and add your cup of ice water to it. Take a fine mesh sieve and pour your milk mixture through it, and into the bowl of ice water. Cover bowl and place in your freezer for the next four hours. After 4 hours in the freezer, take out and serve.

Nutritional Information per Serving

Calories: 328

Total Fat: 27 g

Saturated Fat: 19 g

Cholesterol: 138 mg

Total Carbs: 16 g

Chai Infused Chocolate Pots de Creme

A true classic! This Chai Infused Chocolate Pots de Crème are the cream of the crop!

Prep Time: 25 minutes

Passive Time: 20 minutes

Cook Time: 0 minutes

Total Time: 4 hours

Here are the exact ingredients:

1 cup of coconut milk

3-inch cinnamon stick, crushed

2 tsp crushed cardamom pods

½ tsp whole crushed peppercorns

¼ cup of honey

4 eggs

4 ounces of chopped, unsweetened chocolate

1 tsp of vanilla

Instructions:

Pour your cup of coconut milk into a large saucepan, followed by your crushed 3-inch cinnamon stick, your 2 tsp of crushed cardamom pods, and your ½ tsp of whole crushed peppercorns. Set the burner on high and allow the ingredients to cook for about 15 minutes. Next, strain your mixture through a fine mesh sieve and into a mixing bowl. Throw away any excess spices in the pan, before returning the milk mixture to the pan.

Now add your ¼ cup of honey, and your 4 eggs to the pan, stir all of these ingredients together well as they cook over the next 5 minutes. Turn off your burner and add your tsp of vanilla, followed by your 4 ounces of chopped, unsweetened chocolate. Sir vigorously before pouring mixture into pot de crème cups. Finally, place a cover over them, and place in the fridge. Chill for four hours before serving.

Nutritional Information per Serving

Calories: 211

Total Fat: 18 g

Saturated Fat: 13 g

Cholesterol: 92 mg

Total Carbs: 13 g

Cashew Truffles

Whether on the Paleo Challenge or not—everyone loves their Cashew Truffles! Try this recipe!

Prep Time: 30 min

Passive Time: 1 hour and 25 min

Cook Time: 8 min

Total Time: 2 hours and 3 min

Here are the exact ingredients:

8 ounces of unsweetened chocolate

2 tablespoons of coconut oil

½ cup of canned unsweetened coconut milk

¼ cup of maple syrup

1 tsp of vanilla

¾ cup of whole raw cashews

¼ tsp of sea salt

Instructions:

To get started, put your 8 ounces of unsweetened chocolate, and your 2 tablespoons of coconut oil into a large mixing bowl and stir the ingredients together. Get out a medium sized saucepan and add your ½ cup of unsweetened coconut milk, cook for five minutes and then drizzle it over your chocolate mixture in the mixing bowl. Cover the bowl and place it in your refrigerator, letting it cool for 45 minutes.

While your chilling your chocolate in the fridge, set your oven for 350 degrees. Now take out a medium sized baking pan and add your ¾ cup of raw cashews to the pan. Place in the oven and bake for about 10 minutes, taking it out a couple of times to stir while it cooks. Once cooked transfer your cashews to a separate plastic container and set them to the side for a moment.

Now, going back to your chocolate mixture in the fridge, after it has finished chilling for 45 minutes, take it out and begin to cut it up into 35 individual pieces. Now get out a blender and add your cashews to it, pulsing the two or three times. Pour these over your apportioned truffles. Let the truffles sit at room temps for about a half hour, and serve when ready.

Nutritional Information per Serving

Calories: 69

Total Fat: 6 g

Saturated Fat: 4 g

Cholesterol: 0 mg

Total Carbs: 4 g

Chapter 6: Paleo Soups, Salads, and Sides

Besides regular meals, Paleo offers up quite a few interesting combinations of soups, salads, and sides. The recipes presented in this chapter go well with just about any meal you've got planned. Try them all!

Paleo Avocado Chili Butter

Refined, delicate, and tasteful! Paleo Avocado Chili Butter is a Paleolithic side you won't soon forget! Make it and keep it for when you need it!

Prep Time: 3 min

Passive Time: 0 min

Cook Time: 0 min

Total Time: 3 min

Here are the exact ingredients:

½ cup of chopped avocado

¼ cup of chopped red chili

1 tsp of coriander powder

¼ cup of lime juice

Instructions:

Add the ½ cup of chopped avocado, and ¼ cup of chopped red chili, followed by the ¼ cup of lime juice to a food processor, and press "liquify". After about 1 minute, tur it off, and pour the liquid contents into a medium sized mixing bowl. Sprinkle your tsp of coriander powder on top, stir briefly and serve.

Nutritional Information per Serving

Calories: 70

Total Fat: 4 g

Saturated Fat: 1 g

Cholesterol: 0 mg

Total Carbs: 4 g

Korean Mushroom Soup

A striking combination of tofu, mushrooms, and soy sauce! This Korean Mushroom Soup will make your day!

Prep Time: 5 min

Passive Time: 0 min

Cook Time: 23 min

Total Time: 28 min

Here are the exact ingredients:

½ cup of chopped shiitake mushrooms

¼ cup of olive oil

2 cups of water

½ cup of chopped button mushrooms

1 tablespoon of chopped garlic

½ cup of chopped scallion

2 cups of chicken broth

1 cup of chopped tofu

1 tablespoon of soy sauce

1 tsp of salt

1 tsp of black pepper

Instructions:

Put your ½ cup of shiitake mushrooms, followed by your 2 cups of water into a large plastic, microwave safe container, and microwave for about 8 minutes. Next, take your ¼ cup of olive oil and place it into a medium sized saucepan, on a burner set for medium-high heat. Now add your ½ cup of chopped shiitake mushrooms to the pan and allow them to cook for about 10 minutes, briefly stirring the mushrooms into the oil as they cook.

Follow this by adding your ½ cup of chopped button mushrooms, your 1 tablespoon of chopped garlic, your ½ cup of chopped scallion, your cup of chopped tofu, and your 2 cups of chicken broth. Let these cook for another 5 minutes. Turn your burner off, and marinate the ingredients with your tablespoon of soy sauce, your 1 tsp of salt, and your 1 tsp of black pepper. Serve when ready.

Nutritional Information per Serving

Calories: 249

Total Fat: 12 g

Saturated Fat: 2 g

Cholesterol: 87 mg

Total Carbs: 17 g

<u>*Paleo Pork Salad*</u>

Loaded with pork, eggs, and greens, this salad is good any time of the day!

Prep Time: 3 min

Passive Time: 0 min

Cook Time: 7 min

Total Time: 10 min

Here are the exact ingredients:

2 eggs

7 strips of bacon

2 cups shredded lettuce

Instructions:

First, get out a large serving bowl and deposit your 2 cups of shredded lettuce. Put this to the side for a moment. Place a large frying pan on your stove, with the burner set to medium-high heat. Lay out your 7 strips of bacon in the pan and cook for 5 minutes. Once your 5 minutes are up, remove your bacon from the pan, and lay them out on a napkin or clean towel to absorb the grease.

Add your 2 eggs to the pan, stirring them vigorously as they cook over the next 2 minutes, before turning off the burner. Now empty your eggs out on top of your shredded lettuce in the serving bowl. Follow this by laying out your 7 slices of bacon on top of the egg/lettuce mixture. You can now serve up your Paleo Pork Salad whenever you are ready.

Nutritional Information per Serving

Calories: 389

Total Fat: 12 g

Saturated Fat: 7 g

Cholesterol: 33 mg

Total Carbs: 2 g

<u>*Sweet Fries n' Ketchup*</u>

Roasted sweet potato fries marinated with garlic and ketchup! These Sweet Fries are always a party favorite!

Prep Time: 10 minutes

Passive Time: 0 min

Cook Time: 30 min

Total Time: 40 min

Here are the exact ingredients:

1 and ½ pounds of sweet potatoes

2 tablespoons of olive oil

¾ tsp of sea salt

¼ tsp of black pepper

3 tablespoons, chopped onion

¼ cup of chopped garlic

¼ cup of agave-sweetened ketchup

Instructions:

Set your oven to 450 degrees. While your oven heats up, get out a cutting board and cut your 1 and ½ pounds of sweet potatoes and cut them into ½ inch thick slices. Place your freshly cut potato slices on a large cooking sheet. Drizzle the sweet potatoes with 1 of your tablespoons of olive oil, followed by a sprinkling over your ¾ tsp of sea salt, and ¼ tsp of black pepper. Place your cooking sheet into the oven, and allow it to cook for 30 minutes.

As the sweet potato fries cook, get out a small saucepan and add your 3 tablespoons of chopped onion, and your ¼ cup of chopped garlic. Set the burner on high heat and stir the ingredients for 2 minutes as they cook. Once cooked, turn the burner off, and add your ¼ cup of agave-sweetened ketchup to the mix, stirring everything together well. As soon as your sweet potato fries have finished cooking in the oven, serve them alongside your ketchup mixture. Enjoy!

Nutritional Information per Serving

Calories: 203

Total Fat: 4 g

Saturated Fat: 1 g

Cholesterol: 0 mg

Total Carbs: 41 g

Chunky Guacamole

Whether it's the Super Bowl, a block party or just a weekend with your buddies, this Chunky Guacamole is a side of Paleo goodness that can go the distance!

Prep Time: 15 min

Passive Time: 30 min

Cook Time: 0 min

Total Time 45 min

Here are the exact ingredients:

1 cup of chopped avocadoes

¼ cup of chopped tomatoes

¼ cup of snipped cilantro

¼ cup of chopped red onion

¼ cup of lime juice

¼ cup of chopped jalapenos

¾ tsp of sea salt

¼ cup of chopped garlic

Instructions:

Get a medium sized mixing bowl and add your cup of chopped avocados, followed by your ¼ cup of chopped tomatoes, your ¼ cup of snipped cilantro, your ¼ cup of chopped red onion, your ¼ cup of lime juice, your ¼ cup of chopped jalapenos, your ¾ tsp of sea salt, and your ¼ cup of chopped garlic. Stir these ingredients together before covering them and setting them to the side. Let the ingredients stand at room temperature for 30 minutes. Once your 30 minutes have passed, your Chunky Guacamole is ready to go!

Nutritional Information per Serving

Calories: 71

Total Fat: 6 g

Saturated Fat: 1 g

Cholesterol: 0 mg

Total Carbs: 4 g

Asparagus Salad

An incredibly healthy and satisfying Paleo salad!

Prep Time: 20 min

Passive Time: 30 min

Cook Time: 0 min

Total Time: 0 min

Here are the exact ingredients:

½ cup of chopped red onion

¼ cup of white wine vinegar

1 pound of trimmed asparagus spears

3 cups fresh arugula

2 tablespoons, snipped mint

1 tablespoons olive oil

¼ tsp sea salt

¼ tsp black pepper

Instructions:

Take out a medium sized mixing bowl and add your ½ cup of chopped red onion and your ¼ cup of white wine vinegar. Mix these ingredients together well, before covering the container and putting it to the side. Let this mixture stand at room temperature for about 30 minutes. Meanwhile, get out your pound of trimmed asparagus spears and place them into a large saucepan. Add your cup of water and set the burner for high heat. Cook the asparagus spears for about 5 minutes.

After 5 minutes have passed, turn off the burner, and drain the pan of its water. Now get out a large serving bowl and transfer your cooked asparagus to the bowl. Next, add your 3 cups of arugula and your 2 tablespoons of snipped mint on top of the asparagus. Now, once your onion mixture has stood at room temperature for 30 minutes, pour it over your asparagus mixture in the serving bowl. Follow this up by drizzling your tablespoon of olive oil, your ¼ tsp of sea salt, and your ¼ tsp of black pepper over the ingredients. Serve up your salad when ready.

Nutritional Information per Serving

Calories: 90

Total Fat: 7 g

Saturated Fat: 1 g

Cholesterol: 0 mg

Total Carbs: 5 g

Sea Salt Veggie Chips

Often enough, one of the things that many miss the most when they start the 30-Day Paleo Challenge is their supply of potato chips. But even though standard, heavily processed potato chips are a Paleo no-no, these tasty Sea Salt Veggie Chips are 100% Paleo approved!

Prep Time: 20 min

Passive Time: 8 hours

Cook Time: 0 min

Total Time: 8 hours and 20 min

Here are the exact ingredients:

1 cup of thinly sliced sweet potatoes

1 cup of thinly sliced blue potatoes

1 cup of thinly sliced beets

1 cup of thinly sliced carrots

1 cup of thinly sliced parsnips

½ tsp sea salt

Instructions:

First, get out a large pot of salted water, and place it on a burner set to high heat. Now add your cup of thinly sliced sweet potatoes, your cup of thinly sliced blue potatoes, your cup of thinly sliced beets, your cup of thinly sliced carrots, and your cup of thinly sliced parsnips to the pot. Bring the water to a boil, and boil these ingredients for about 1 minute. Turn off the burner and drain the moisture from all of your veggies with a colander.

Place your drained veggies in a large bowl and evenly distribute your ½ tsp of sea salt over them. After doing this place your salted veggie slices out on dehydrator trays and dehydrate them at 135 degrees for about 8 hours. After 8 hours your Sea Salt Veggie Chips are ready!

Nutritional Information per Serving

Calories: 50

Total Fat: 0 g

Saturated Fat: 0 g

Cholesterol: 0 g

Total Carbs: 12 g

Conclusion: The Best 30 Days of Your Life!

It really is amazing how much your life can change in just 30 days' time. A sustained regimen of Paleo can reboot your body, and your entire state of mind. It may be difficult the first few days of your challenge but you will find after the end of the first week, that you will feel a gradual lift in you spirits. You will notice an extra boost to your overall energy and stamina as you go through your day.

All of the ingredients, recipes, and anecdotal testimony provided in this book, are presented here as guide posts to lead you through your 30-day challenge to make them as pleasant and productive as they can possibly be. Follow the guidelines of this book and you just might find that the month you spend with the Paleo diet was not only manageable, but quite possibly the best 30 days of your life! Thank you for reading!

Made in the USA
Middletown, DE
25 August 2018